The Elevated Life

Living Life Above Circumstance

By A.K. Gray

ISBN: 978-0-578-72656-4

Dedication

This book is dedicated to my children. Roderick, Brian and Kristopher, you have been my pain, fear, joy and my love; the motive in the forefront of my grit and grind. In raising you I have also raised myself, grown up, realized my weaknesses, strength's and capabilities. Love you guys to the core.

To my daughter Niya, there is a river of love for you that flows deeper than words and one day you will understand the depths of it.

Contents

Preface

This book is inspired by Source. You may see many variations throughout the book referencing **the Creator** or **Source**, **God**, **Yahweh**, **Jehovah**, **Infinite Intelligence**, but my opinion is that there is only one Creator with many names.

I am not religious in the traditional sense of the word; I am not a guru, a Buddhist, a yoga master or a psychologist. I am just a girl with inspired vision birthed through life experience, in a relationship with her Creator, and connected to this Universe.

Daily I remain open, mindful, living out this plan with purpose, on purpose, deliberately. My objective is to affect some change and bring some good to others who may have lost hope; yet constantly holding on to my own hopefulness on behalf of the collective.

Forever believing that my words will supply a soothing balm to open wounds and that they will uplift, bring clarity, introspection, and eventually inspiration. Deeply grateful for the opportunity to share this message even if the only life that I touch or am blessed to inspire... is *yours;* even this is more than enough.

The Elevated Life

I

Survival Mode

> *"Let us make man in our image and after our*
> *likeness...and let them have DOMINION over the*
> *earth...be fruitful and multiply"*
> – (GENESIS 1:26– 28, EMPHASIS MINE)

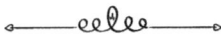

———eeﾒee———

*I*t is difficult finding oneself in unseemly situations. For example, divorce can be one of the most emotionally debilitating setbacks to ever experience. Divorce literally means severance of a union, a breaking of a covenant relationship, the breaking of a vow or promise.

You must understand that divorce, for reasons outside of abuse or adultery, is never one's intention or desire. Usually people marry as an outward expression of their love and solidarity to the commitment of staying together.

I believe that a great, even good marriage requires a lifetime commitment of not only love but also respect for the relationship and each other. Additionally, if there are children incorporated into this unit, conceived from love, there is a stronger, mutual desire to preserve the familial construct of the marriage union. Divorce is a lie when it is promulgated as a "be all, end all" resolution. Even the Creator has stated in the good book that the original plan has always been for the union of the man, and the woman forming a supportive system through which they might create , populate the earth forming our societies, cultures and cultivating diversity.

"...make man (humankind) in our image..." Not only are we gods (*that* is another book topic), but our Unity, strength, and capabilities are magnified when we present a unified front. We are stronger together rather than separate. This is true for any relationship—not just married couples but those in loving, committed relationships without "the paper."

Divorce, separation, breakups, etc.—they are all the same. Severance is severance in any relational context. But shit happens. Even though the severance of a union, the painful remnants of a broken relationship, and a broken dream are all that seem to linger, you will rise above the pain and brokenness.

Divorce is not the only extreme circumstance that could affect our lives negatively. What about loss? Personal, health, financial, or otherwise. These types of circumstances could find us in a place of lack, despair, and confusion.

Imagine working your whole life to build a stable financial future, seemingly doing all the right things by society's standards, following "the rules, then losing it all (the things that determined your self-esteem, value, and worth). Feelings of emptiness result after the loss because you associated all your value and worth with the amassing of things, but no emotional balance.

Or maybe all of your life you have been fed a story of worthlessness and lived through years of abuse, physical or emotional, that have left you functional in some capacity but never fully reaching your highest potential because you are stuck in a belief that was imprinted in your subconscious repeatedly. Conditioning you to a life of repeated failures. These life upsets, contrasting situations, and life-altering events carry with them a load of other contingencies that are the aftereffects of their action.

The list includes trust or trust issues, questionable self-confidence, low self-esteem, fear, despair, depression, guilt, feelings of inferiority, feelings of loss, financial worry, and struggle. It takes a lot to rise above or come back from these kinds of losses. These aftereffects are the tricks, schemes, and lies of the enemy—the enemy that, at the time, may even be ourselves, our very own feelings of despair, fear, and negative self-talk, or things we were taught to believe about ourselves.

Thankfully, your current circumstance is Not the end of your story. We must find the inner resolve to realize that the enemy's plan, the enemy of self, the enemy of love and light, will not prevail.

The Universe's plan is greater, and an intentional shift in thought, feeling, and emotion (followed by inspired action) will be the determining factor of your future happiness. You can do more than just survive any setback; you can thrive.

Learning to live a happy life after any serious loss or traumatic experience takes will, intention, desire, and practicing new thought processes.

Are you willing to do the work to start your life on a new and beautiful adventure of discovery and awakening? The possibilities are endless, but will you set aside your previous way of doing things and do the new work?

There are a couple of things to consider. First are the well-meaning people in our lives.

At times we cannot begin the work of healing, moving on, rebuilding, and becoming whole because we are influenced, both negatively and positively, by external feedback. We then become subjected to making decisions based upon what other people are doing, telling us or suggesting we do. This may not always be in our best interest, especially if the suggestions or feedback are coming from the wrong sources. For instance, oftentimes we have several different people interjecting themselves into our personal business. Specifically, the business of our relationship, finances, and well-being. We end up having him, her, they, mom, dad, cousin, neighbor, and everyone else replaying, commenting, and criticizing the intricacies of our marriage and our relationships. We also receive nostalgic commentary about who we should have or should not have been involved with. Or what about advice and opinions; from those on the outside looking in, about how we handled or should have handled our money or our lives, when they never lived a day in our experience and can't understand our deep feelings and emotions.

They have simply developed their opinions and one-sided vantage point based on a singular perspective that you may have inadvertently alluded to in earlier conversations. Or opinions based upon what they have observed from the outside.

Nonetheless, you get the feedback and pity party support of all of those well-intentioned, uncertified life coaches and self-ordained experts, as well as an earful of their advice. Funny thing is, while being consoled and charitably counseled, you can't help but wonder when these folks became so invested.

Yes, these "experts" tend to be very free and open with advice about what you could have or should have done to keep the relationship, or why you didn't need him, her, or them in the first place. They even go so far as to give you a detailed description of how you should have or should not have handled your money, along with examples of what *they* would have done. Yet again they cannot help but be influenced by, or limited to, their personal experience and bias based on their current mode of thought or feeling. The need to take a side on the issue, may inordinately affect the *unbiased* perspectives of those well intentioned, self-ordained experts. Your loved one's intentionally *objective* opinion could easily become skewed and more *subjective* based on the premise by which it was formulated.

You also get the fear and despair mongers, the pity partiers, and those that support your grief and depressive validation of the loss. Their advice may be motivated solely by their own unresolved issues. Now don't get me wrong. Of course, there is comfort and solace in this attention. It's addictive, soothing even. It allows you to wallow in the hurt and pain of it all with a cheerleader to boot. Effectively being lulled into accepting the mood as your reality, conditioning your mind to think your sulking and sinking into the comforting depths of abandon and disassociation are acceptable.

Well they aren't.

Is it okay to wallow in shit?

That's right; shit, mess, crud, waste. That's how that pain, that grief, that loss feels. Who wants to feel shitty? I don't, and neither should you. It's up to you to want out of this shitty-feeling mess, and you can begin the process of doing that.

First…

» Acknowledge the mess; do not become fixated on or consumed by it.

» Take time to intentionally quiet your mind.

» Reflect on all the good in your life Now.

» FORGIVE and let go.

Acknowledge the mess…. Acknowledging the mess puts it in perspective. You are going to look that shit squarely in its face and see what the hell is really going on. No rationalization here, no beating yourself up about it, no blaming the world, another person, society. None of that. Hell, it is what it is, even if you, or all those mentioned in the previous sentence, were a contributing factor. That does not matter though. How would you benefit from criticizing yourself or anyone else anyway? Especially over events that occurred but cannot be undone? There is no benefit, no forward movement, healing, or rebuilding available to you in that course of action or thinking.

Now let us get back to handling this shit.

Just look. Have an honest observation. You will not be here long; however, look at everything that comprises that shit. Realistically. See it for what it is. Some of it was you, some of it him, some of it her, some of it us. Some of it is simply the result of our own thinking.

Maybe our justification for wallowing might just be that we had a cheating spouse or significant other, an abusive (verbal or physical) partner. Perhaps we could have made a different business or financial decision that would have afforded a different outcome. Maybe if we voted differently. Maybe if we took better preventative measures. Maybe we were just stupid. Or maybe all the negative things we have been fed about ourselves, our economy, or our lives, for however long we have listened, really is the truth, and we will really never amount to, be, or do anything greater than mediocrity and struggle.

We tend to feel like either the level of betrayal or our negative surmising justifies our wallowing in a grievous, depressive, self-deprecating state.

Nope…Not justified; it is still shit. Bullshit actually.

Nonetheless, we still find ourselves thinking about what could have been done differently. How could this shit have been curtailed, missed, contained…? Hell, avoided? Panic about what the hell we're going to do now kicks in. Should you go back to your lover, beg forgiveness at the job you lost or career that failed, find a way to latch on to some other presumed security? All the while compromising your happiness, inner peace, mental or physical well-being because you are afraid to turn the corner of the "what's next" possibilities?

We cannot nurse the negative aspects or contributing factors. The "why me," or maybe "I should or shouldn't have." Our mind will never absolve the alleged perpetrator or endless excuses and wailings of "why me." Our perspective must shift.

Whether it's us, them, or it, the list will go on in our minds. Constantly replaying the negativity until we find a probable, valid, supporting premise and justification for our angst. Horrible nasty truths perhaps. Nonetheless, these considerations continually stagnate block us from obtaining peace, letting go, and moving forward to solution.

It's even more challenging to move forward when your reasoning is dependent upon the nature or cause of the issue, divorce, breakup, severance, or other tangible loss. Yet again, that's just you arguing for your limitations and justifying your wallowing. You think the seemingly justifiable reasons of why shit happened give you more right to have a pity party and stay there nursing it?

Uhhh. No.

Look at it, grieve if you must; but then pick yourself up and get back to your life.

Hard truth to see, difficult concept to embrace, but completely doable.

The reality is that shit has now become waste that has been eliminated from your life. You've acknowledged it, felt every part of it, but you *Don't* live there in it. It's gross. Gross mentally, emotionally, and sometimes physically.

That was not your best life, but there Absolutely is opportunity to cultivate better and begin planting the seeds of a greater future Now.

That's it. That's all. Get up from there if it is your intention to feel better. Get past this, and grow.

Let's keep it moving.

What is real right now, in this present moment, is that the process of elimination has occurred allowing for the removal of all that shit. No matter the cause, the path is clear for newness. Once we observe our shit, our mess, the results our thinking has produced, and see it for the shitty crap it really is in this present moment, we can observe it, grieve it, get over it, and let it go because we're not coming back here to revisit it.

Forward movement only.

Our system has basically had a cleansing. Anything *good* left from that mess has been absorbed, and you get to keep that part.

Good? Good? From shit? Yes. Good. That positive stuff that's left over after the process of elimination (*a series of actions tending to a desired result*) has completed its purpose.

The positive "stuff" that I refer to, are those lessons you learned about yourself. The lessons that helped you to better define exactly what you *Do* want in a love relationship, your finances, your life, or your health and wholeness. The experiences, situations, or circumstances that caused you to come face-to-face with knowing exactly what you Don't want.

Contemplatively regard the context of this analogy. When you get rid of shit physiologically, you are eliminating waste and everything else that is Not essentially good or needed for the body. Shitty life circumstances are comparable. But the good that can be extracted from a negative circumstance or life upset *is* that *good that was gained,* resulting from elimination of the old, nasty, unhealthy shit. The good stuff that, with unbiased consideration and a positive outlook, may help awaken thoughts of hope in the possibility of a better, happier, more fulfilled you.

Just a flicker of hope is all you need to begin to shift. Just a tiny spark to ignite a flame in your heart so intense that subconsciously you Invite the beginnings of your best life into manifestation by a single thought: *what if I could have,* or *what if I could accomplish,* or *what would the best version of my life look like if I...?* That one seed of unspoken faith causing the Universe to hear and begin putting things in motion to bring T_{HAT} kind of *good* smack...dab into the middle of your existence.

You can begin again and allow your latter to be greater than what has passed.

Take time to intentionally quiet the mind…Taking time to intentionally quiet your mind is necessary after cleansing from unwanted mess. You have grieved the loss, rehearsed all the wrongs, rights, should haves, could haves. Finally, now you are at a place where you realize and accept that there actually was some "residual" good stuff that rose to the surface after the mess and, with it, hope for better.

To build on that hope so it becomes a focal point that affects your thinking, changes your mindset and strengthens your positive resolve, you will need to take time to quiet your mind—regularly.

Remember now; there is work involved in this, but the work is easy, and it's beneficial. There is a process (*a series of actions tending to a desired result*). When I say quiet your mind, it's just that. Practiced focus on being still mentally. Focused emotion, focused thought. Ceasing the momentum of a mind all over the place, running insidiously on negativity, thoughts of doubt, despair, sadness, or fear.

Practicing stillness gets you prepared for new thought processes. Allows you to hear from Source (*God, the Universe, Infinite Intelligence—many names but only one Creator*) and connect with the truth of who you are In your true potential. It's an opportunity for connection to higher consciousness that not only restores you but elevates your thinking and reprograms your mind. Think of it as a reformation or readjustment. Reprogram to match the frequency that is the same as the frequency of your predestined best self and your best purposed life. That's why you're here.

Oftentimes, we don't even have a clue who our best self is or how to tap into our Higher Conscious. We've never met him or her. Never even taken time to consider the deeper part of who we are, to think about or imagine what our best life could be like. We've not allowed ourselves to connect at that level. We don't even know how. We just accept whatever thought comes without question. How could we ever have a clue about what we as individuals would define as our best if we've never taken time to imagine the possibilities? Mentally, spiritually, physically, materially.

No, we've been too busy playing follow the leader, following a social stigma of the way to "be." Influenced subconsciously through adopted culture, social norms, religion, power agendas, and the like.

We accept that what someone says or does to us determines the truth about ourselves or our circumstances. When the narrative is negative, often we are accepting what we see and what we hear or looking at our present circumstances, consciously making determinations based on that obscured observation, and allowing our perception to conform to its inaccuracies. Inaccuracies because we are only observing and processing "what is", without realizing the "what is" is temporary and subject to change.

We do this accepting passively, without regard. Not realizing the consequence of negative emotional thought processes. It happens in our minds first because we don't challenge the thought or "check it" at the onset of its development or suggestion.

Any conscious, accepted, despairing thought about a circumstance, situation, or event that is solely motivated by what is right in front of us or what is going on at that very moment, without challenging the validity of that thought against its opposition, pretty much makes us slaves to the outcome of that focused momentum.

We succumb to the opposing view of "what is." We formulate and accept a thought or opinion about it and just accept what we see as our reality in its finality. Simply settling for whatever the circumstance dictates without realizing we... Do...Not...Have...To...We are Not victims.

We have been given the ability to transform our lives. We can start by first taking control of our mind. Corralling the sometimes incessantly foolish, aberrantly suggestive, occasionally paranoid, mostly uncontrolled, all-over-the-place thoughts. Instead, practice reconditioning. Steering the mind to thoughts of our specific desires in opposition of *it (our mind)*, using us, on a daily basis, with circular, repetitive thoughts; flip-flopping emotions, moods, and eventually the outcomes we manifest.

Stop The Noise and get deliberate in your thought process. Get quiet and let the Universe speak truth to you. Connect with your higher, inner self, connect with

Gods originally defined and created you. The rest of the plan will continue to be revealed as you learn to listen for Divine inspiration and direction. Everything will begin to fall into place almost effortlessly as you learn to release the stress, strain, emotion, and unrealistic control or lack thereof.

Be still and quiet your mind; begin to develop new thought processes. You can begin to basically bend reality in your favor and *create* the life you genuinely want instead of letting the adverse circumstances of life steer and lead whichever way it wants by default. Don't you know that you are the "Master of your own ship?" Don't give away your creative power to happenstance, circumstance, or situation. Grab those oars and let's move in the direction of your desires.

Exercise I

Find a quiet place where you will not be disturbed or interrupted. Get comfortable but not so comfortable that you fall asleep. It's important that you stay aware. You can either lie down on your back or sit in a comfortable chair, or in a quiet place on your floor with a small, semi-firm cushion. If you are sitting, sit with body relaxed and upright. More formal methods of quieting the mind in the form of meditation suggest that proper posture be practiced. The following listed postures consist of three suggested sitting options and one Mudra (finger/hand positioning/gesture):

1. The Lotus Option: Left foot on top of the right thigh and right foot on top of the left thigh.

2. The Half Lotus Option: Put just one foot (left foot or right foot) on top of the free thigh (left or right) and leave the

uncrossed foot beneath the thigh of the foot in the half lotus.

3. The Crisscrossed Option: Simply sit with legs crisscrossing each other with feet beneath each thigh or crossed at the ankles directly in front of you.

4. Chin Mudra (hand position) Option: Chin means consciousness in Sanskrit, and Mudra means gesture. This Mudra is another way to connect to inner self more deeply. It helps to ground you in awareness and raises energy. Feel free to incorporate this Mudra at your discretion, or not.

Using both hands, hold the thumb and index fingers together lightly. They need only to touch without exerting any pressure. The remaining three fingers are pointing out and as straight as possible. The hands can then be placed on the thighs, palms up. This is a hand positioning option to consider when practicing quieting the mind. This is not a directive or requirement for achieving the intended result. Your hands can be folded in your lap, resting on your thighs, or however you feel comfortable.

Wherever/however you are comfortable is key. Keep in mind the options listed above are just that—suggested options. They are Not requirements for quieting the mind. This guide neither endorses nor promotes Buddhism. The philosophy is familiar, appreciated, and respected but not practiced in this book.

Now let's begin.

Close your eyes and breathe in deeply through your nose; feel your belly slowly growing like a balloon, filling up with air as you inhale. Slightly part your lips as you exhale if you'd like or simply keep your mouth closed and gently exhale through the nose, really feeling the breath leave your body. Take another slow, deep breath in. Hold that breath in for an extra second then gently exhale. As you do so, feel your body start to loosen up. Take in another deep breath, paying attention to the expansion in your chest and belly as you do so, hold it for a second, and, as you gently exhale, release all thoughts of anxiety, tension, anger, and stress. Feel the feeling of your entire body letting go. Take in another deep breath, feeling every muscle in your body begin to relax. As you gently exhale, release and let go of any thoughts of anger or worry and feel every muscle in your body, from your neck, shoulders, back, thighs, fingertips to your toes, completely and totally relax. Take several deeper breaths in and out and focus on your breathing. Quietly listen to the rhythm of your breathing.

You are quieting your mind. Just breathe. No forced thought. If you find yourself beginning to think about the day's events or things to be done, just acknowledge the thought and gently redirect yourself to your breathing. Try to get to a place of completely no thought, detachment from everything going on around you. You will ultimately connect with Higher Conscious, and an overwhelming sense of release and a type of spiritual ecstasy can be experienced. At this point, stay settled, become aware of the now moment, and simply allow the Universe to unfold for you. Just relax, breathe and open to receive whatever downloads that come from Higher Conscious. Just be. In this place is the beginning of complete inner peace, awakening, and new thought processes.

I recommend fifteen-minutes-a-day of getting still and quieting your mind, at the beginning of the day before daily activity begins, and again (if possible) in the evenings to reconnect. As you make a daily practice of this, you may find that you love it so much, it becomes a habitual, necessary part of your daily routine. Your fifteen minutes could easily turn to twenty or thirty. I don't recommend more than thirty-minutes-per-session; it might make you top heavy... heady. Let having *total* mind, body, and soul *balance* be your endeavor.

Finally….

Reflect on all the good…Reflect on all the Good in your life Now. There is so much that is good here and now. You have taken deliberate action to positively affect the mental trajectory of change in your thinking that will directly move your life in the direction you want things to go.

Good.

You have made a conscious, deliberate, decision that you will no longer passively allow your thoughts to govern how you feel when faced with what may look like variant contrast.

Incredibly good.

You know and understand that what is seen is temporary and subject to revision, depending on your thoughts, perspectives, and next moves.

Exceptionally good.

You have begun to understand that the deliberate monitoring, deliberate directing of your thoughts is your innate power to self-regulate your emotions. You are Not a victim.

Sooo damn good!

You have been given the ability to create your reality and transform your life.

Powerfully good!

You are truly at a turning point in your life, an awakening. You can make it Whatever you want it to be.

Taking time to think about all the good things in your life right now forces your mind to shift its focus, and that shift will also affect your feeling state, your emotions.

Say to yourself or aloud:

I am blessed. I am truly blessed. I know it and believe it to my core. I am reticently reactive to contrast, knowing that even in contrast I am becoming more resilient and prepared for the amazing changes unfolding in my life. my possibilities are endless. I Declare and allow these possibilities to be revealed, confirmed, increasingly clarified to me as I take time to get still and quiet my mind. I will remember who I am in my potential.

II

Change Your Thinking by Changing What You Believe

"Your life is a reflection of your thoughts. If you change your thinking you change your life."

–BRIAN TRACY

———— ꙮꙮ ————

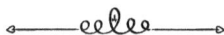

*M*any people question themselves and perpetuate a negative, practiced belief or unhealthy, inappropriate action response when faced with situations in life that are perceived negatively or that go in a direction that is different than desired. An outcome that develops that is contrary to that which we've expected. As a result, we oftentimes begin telling ourselves things like "There is something wrong with me."

We tend to question, who we are, or why our current circumstance is raw and unfulfilling. Or why our life appears to be unraveling.

Constantly asking ourselves, "Why did this happen?" Or, "Why does this kind of shit always happen to me? There must be something wrong with me. Why can't I get things right? Damn, I failed again!" And so on and so on. You can probably think of a million reasons to mentally beat yourself up about; especially in a failed situation or outcome, that simply just aren't the complete Truth. They are your *feeling* of a truth based on what you believe. What you're rehearsing is what your current, practiced beliefs have conditioned your subconscious to believe as truth.

It is the thought base that your mind resorts to in the event there is a situation, circumstance, or crisis. Any kind of contrast that arises and makes you feel there is no other explanation for it but what You did wrong. It's all your fault. It's a disaster.

These types of thoughts or reactions stem from our past or some similarly experienced situation we've encountered before and have an embedded recollective response that activates subconsciously as our protective resolve.

Basically, negative thought patterns can be a practiced defense cultivated by your past reactions implanted in the subconscious as the way to respond over and over again in similar types of situations.

For some of us, the contributing factor may have even been the familial construct we were exposed to growing up. What we've seen or heard in response or reaction to...trouble or challenge, i.e., contrast. What others have repetitively told us while growing up as children or the people, situations, and conditions we were influenced by. These things shaped and conditioned what we feel about ourselves today. Not only how we feel about ourselves but also how we choose to respond to contrast in our lives. Not only being repetitively exposed to negative conversation but also seeing our parents, loved ones, or care givers respond to certain situations that also helped to, by example, condition our thinking to respond to stressful situations in a certain comparable manner. Just watching how situations were dealt with in our day-to-day may be the only way we know how to cope, which means it will influence our fight or flight response in dealing with our current mess. How we have been taught to protect ourselves basically.

Whether our observed remedy was to self-medicate, respond aggressively, deflect onto others by being abusive either verbally or physically, withdraw, or internalize and beat up on ourselves with the negative self-talk.

To begin to attack yourself and question who you are in a negative light is a trick of the enemy and an attack on your character and self-esteem. Do not believe these lies. It's just an adverse effect of the situation, but don't be ruled by it and do not be consumed by thoughts and rationalizations about what you could have done to make things better.

You know why? It's a waste of time, thought, and energy to dwell on what could have been or what you could have done differently. The situation, circumstance, or issue—whatever it is or was—is final at this point. Beating yourself up about the whys and how imperfect you think you are is not productive, nor can it resolve any earlier condition. It's okay to let yourself off the hook. Chill a little. Be okay with not being okay and Not feeling badly about yourself for this current shift in your life. Start changing your belief by changing your thinking. Think and realize that you are a child of God, the Creator, Source, Infinite Intelligence. No mistake was made when you were created. In every element, everything, every characteristic, every move you make, every thought, every decision, every action made by you, is *No* surprise in the Creator's eyes. Before the beginning of time, you were known. In every circumstance and situation, you are enough just the way you are. Practice this belief every day.

It's time to pick up the broken pieces of what is left of you and forge ahead. God, the Universe, Source, the Creator has a plan for you that is better than what you thought you had before. In order to hear it, get your mind clear. Get clarity and get understanding.

Shake yourself and wake the fuck up.

Remove the negative clutter and negative self-talk; open your ears and listen for the words of truth. Open and dry your eyes; prepare to write the new vision. Unbind your heart to new beliefs about yourself and your power. You are a powerful creator, and, by your thoughts and beliefs, you create your reality.

What you have already manifested is, of course, a result of what your thoughts, beliefs, and self-talk have created, but let it be your catalyst for change and not your punishment or opportunity for martyrdom.

Everything that we live in this moment is a thought manifested. That thought came alive because of a strong belief. That belief was promulgated by repetition and strong emotion. Look back over your life; see the material things around you, the people in your life, even the current circumstances both good and bad. Closely observe and consider. You will come to the realization of *Your* created reality. You are in the midst of the life that you—consciously or subconsciously, on purpose or by default—created.

Remember the time when you believed something very intensely? Your thoughts and imaginations formulated opinions, images in your mind, visions, wished opportunities, affirmations, or negations. A day, week, month, or year later, what you envisioned occurs. Or maybe that person you were thinking of or desirous for communication with comes into your life or makes some kind of contact with you! That's how strong belief, repetitively practiced as thought, manifests a person, thing, circumstance, or situation.

Establishing purpose in thought, changing outdated, rigid, controlling beliefs, is a necessary action in changing the course of our lives.

Not possible, you say? What about destiny? Preordination theories? Or what about the paths of our lives that are already drawn, invisibly mapped out for us. The course that is inevitable in its becoming. Or perhaps you take on the attitude *"Que sera sera / Whatever will be will be / The future is not ours to see / Que sera sera."* It is what it is; it can't be changed.

Bullshit!

The future may not be ours to see, but I'm damn sure we have the power to steer the direction of what's to come by energetically, deliberately thinking on, focusing on, and contemplating the outcome we want.

Everything contrary to your believing and understanding that thoughts create reality or that your life is left to chance and happenstance that you do not have the ability or power to affect; are simply rehearsed convictions. Beliefs you've been taught, picked up from somewhere, felt strongly about, internalized, and practiced repetitiously with an emotional attachment. Inadvertently these became your adopted truths.

Thank goodness change is inevitable. It's coming whether we want it or not. That and time are the only things we don't have control over, and that's okay. If you are reading this book, today you have *time*; and, although we cannot control change, we can definitely manipulate it to our advantage.

Change and time allow for opportunity. The seasons change over time, and there is a falling away, a pruning, a shift that gives way to newness. This is a natural process of nature itself. What makes you think that in the seasons of your own life—as intricately designed and as detailed as God has made you—that you should be sitting on your ass, lamenting what was or currently is? Simply waiting for the winds to sway and move you hither and thither on a whim of chance yet never being proactive in the course of your life. Just taking whatever life presents to you. That's not what you were made for. You were created for more. To live life abundantly. To live life on purpose, with purpose.

The Creator's plans for you are good. "'For I know the plans I have for you,' declares the Lord, 'plans to prosper you and not to harm you, plans to give you hope and a future.'" (Jeremiah 29:11, NIV) Why not bridge your efforts with Divine synchronicity?

Allow those good plans. Co-create with Source, whose Purpose for you is hope, prosperity, and a bright future. Partner up. Get tuned in and tap into Higher Consciousness. Activate and stir up deep states of intuition and creativity.

HEAR, in the innermost parts of you; with your heart, the plans for your life. Your very own ***DIVINELY*** ordained desires being birthed into tangible existence. There are deep desires that can only begin to surface as you go deeper introspectively to discover the blueprint of your purpose. The blueprint imbedded in your subconscious, lying dormant since before the beginning of your physical existence, waiting for you to awaken to higher conscious—ask for it, write the plan, and believe it is done. Stop disallowing your abundant life with so much focused thought on what's gone wrong.

Become an active co-creator in the designing of a happy, whole, fulfilling life that is your real truth. Focus on what you <u>Want</u>, not what is unwanted.

Focus energy on what's wanted. See your reality; feel the feeling of That reality...that's how you start.

Wouldn't it be nice to tap into beliefs and thoughts that begin to redirect your current path? That steer your life into new, exciting, healthy, happy, and prosperous directions?

Hell yeah!

Thoughts do become things and manifest in our current reality. Their foundation and content are given ammunition, energy, and strength through our very own beliefs. Therefore, it is vitally important that we manage our thoughts so that they are not running rampant and unconfined in negativity or unpredictability.

Use and direct your thoughts, your mind. Do not let your thoughts, your mind, use you.

Consider your thoughts because "*as a man thinketh, so is he.*" You Are and you Produce what you think. Thoughts are energy and become things in your personage, your circumstances, and situations. Everything that makes up your life is derived from a thought.

What are you saying to yourself each day? Consider your thoughts.

From the moment you awaken each morning, throughout the day, to the moment you lie down again to sleep, practice being intentional about your focus. You should be thinking intentionally about how you want to experience the day. As it unfolds, Source takes that intention and expounds it exponentially, exceedingly, abundantly, above your desired expectation, surprising you with sheer delight and bliss throughout the day.

At that point, in that state of positive momentum and good energy, any number of manifestations are sure to become a part of your experience and will be for your ultimate good. All of that possibility results because you exercised due diligence in intentionally setting the tone of your day. From the time you open your eyes to greet the new day, aim to practice this intention continually until it is habit. Do not wake up and just let your mind run rampant, replaying all the negatives of yesterday or the contemptible possibilities of the current day.

No.

With deliberate intent, You decide to take your conscious power back, and, as the powerful co-creator that you Are, you set the tone of your day.

Did you feel that? Did you feel the energy of happy momentum as you read those words in the last paragraph? Feel it. That's where you need to be at the beginning of the day; as soon as you wake up, be on purpose. As you repetitively practice being on purpose and intentional each morning, the frequency of your vibration begins to change and align with all that the Universe has available for you. Additionally, consciousness begins to inform the subconscious of how things will go moving forward, and consciousness is validated in this shift by the creations that are gradually manifesting. Then things start getting

53

really exciting as you see your desires that were at first just thoughts and imaginations, turning into things and appearing in your life that you created --- Intentionally.

It's an amazing phenomenon. Like magic, but it's not; it's just you exercising your creative power to transform your life.

There is nothing wrong with you, beloved. "You are fearfully and wonderfully made."

Exercise II: Intention Hour

1. Set your alarm the night before for at least an hour earlier than your normal wake-up time. If you'd like, have a small pen and notepad or journal nearby to record thoughts and affirmations that you can reflect on the following day or even throughout the day, if you feel so inclined. When you awake in the morning, do the following: Lying down or sitting up,

greet the day with an immediate "Thank you" and a smile. Feel thankful. Make the feeling of thankfulness as intense as you want it to be. Think about how thankful you are simply to have a new day of brand- new possibilities. This takes about five minutes of your intention hour.

2. Grab your notepad/journal and pen. Write down (at the very least) five things that you are grateful for this morning (whether you have them now or want to experience them; either way, write in the present tense). Spend about ten-to-fifteen minutes on this. Example: I Am happy and thankful Now that I Am... healthy, and whole.

3. Lying down or sitting up, greet the day with an immediate "Thank you" and a

smile. Feel thankful. Make the feeling of thankfulness as intense as you want it to be. Think about how thankful you are simply to have a new day of brand-new possibilities. This takes about five minutes of your intention hour.

4. Grab your notepad/journal and pen. Write down (at the very least but as many as you want) five things that you are grateful for this morning (whether you have them now or want to experience them; either way, write in the present tense). Spend about ten-to-fifteen minutes on this. Example:

a) I Am so happy and thankful Now that I Am…happy, healthy, and whole.

b) I Am so happy and thankful Now that I have...a wonderful, loving, supportive partner.

c) I Am so happy and thankful for... healthy, delicious food to eat.

d) I Am so happy and thankful Now that I Am...prosperous and successful in every endeavor.

5. Next, let's take fifteen minutes to quiet the mind and incorporate the meditation exercise we practiced in Chapter I. Close your eyes and breathe in deeply through your nose; feel your belly slowly growing like a balloon, filling up with air as you inhale. Slightly part your lips as you exhale if you would like or simply keep your mouth closed and gently exhale through the nose, really feeling the breath leave your body. Take another slow, deep

breath in. Hold that breath in for an extra second then gently exhale. As you do so, feel your body start to loosen up.

Take in another deep breath, paying attention to the expansion in your chest and belly as you do so, hold it for a second, and, as you gently exhale, release all thoughts of anxiety, tension, anger, and stress. Feel the feeling of your entire body letting go. Take in another deep breath, feeling every muscle in your body begin to relax. As you gently exhale, release and let go of any thoughts of anger or worry and feel every muscle in your body, from your neck, shoulders, back, thighs, fingertips to your toes, completely and totally relax. Take several deeper breaths in and out and focus on your breathing. Quietly listen to the rhythm of your breathing. You are quieting your mind. Just breathe. No forced thought. If you find yourself beginning to think about the day's events or things to be done, just acknowledge the thought and gently redirect yourself to your breathing. Try to get to a place of completely no thought, detachment from everything going on in and around you, except your awareness of only Now and your breathing. In this place is the beginning of complete inner peace, awakening, and new thought processes.

6. Take about fifteen minutes to make your affirmations and verbally declare the day. Being intentional about setting the tone. You can either speak the declaration or write it down in your journal or note pad, or both. Your declaration sets the tone of your day. Daily practice,

frequency, and feeling produce results, but you must at least start the process. In making your affirmations be sure to have the following:

a) Concise (to-the-point) choice of positive words at the beginning of each affirmation. Ex: "Today is the beginning of a phenomenal day full of amazing possibilities. I choose to own this day. It will be productive and successful." Or "I love my life. This day is going to be filled with endless possibilities, and each possibility is working out in my favor." Or "Today there is absolutely nothing that I cannot do."

b) Feel the feeling of high energy and momentum as you write and speak your declaration. Feeling the words you speak and adding emotion behind it creates energy, and energy is magnetic, drawing all things alike unto itself.

c) Finally, form a mental image of yourself realizing the declaration. Visualize yourself smiling and experiencing the declarations you made. The tone of the day has been set, and It Is Good.

The key thing to remember in creating your affirmations and making your declarations is that your subconscious knows and is aware of who you really are, how you really think, and your familiar vibration. Make your affirmations believable truths so that you work with your mind's current level of belief and not against it. It will buck at you. You must gradually and repetitively nudge and reshape old beliefs until they yield and conform to the new. You can gauge your believable truth by how you feel when you speak it. In the center of your chest, in your heart area, does it get tight or feel easy? If it's easy, you got it. If tight or uncomfortable, change the affirmation wording. Sometimes past energy belief affects present energy belief, and changing that belief is a gradual, repetitive process that will enable future affirmations to more effectively produce the outcomes we want. This will be addressed further in a future chapter.

III

It's All Energy and Vibrational Frequency

"Everything is energy and that's all there is to it. Match the frequency of the reality you want, and you cannot help but get that reality. It can be no other way. This is not philosophy. This is physics."

–Albert Einstein

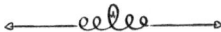

———eeℓee———

"…This is not philosophy. This is physics." Einstein makes the definite distinction between the two as they relate to energy and frequency. This is one of my favorite quotes. However, I do believe there *is* a correlation between the physics of energy on frequency and the philosophical aspect.

The physics affords us the scientific premise for matter and energy and how frequency brings it together. This same premise transfers over into the reality of our lives and our existence as we consider philosophically how the concept of physics transfers over to mental energy, thought process, and creation of a manifested thing. By matching the frequency of it (it being the thing or the reality we want to manifest).

We are matter, substance, and energy. Because of this, we have the capability of transcending the laws of mechanical physics and matching the frequency of a desired reality.

Do you realize that you have the ability to self-regulate the flow of any outcome? Through the validations in these outcomes, consciousness informs itself by the creations that are manifested, good or bad, positive or negative.

The philosophical aspect of this concept considers what steps, what mental processes are necessary in or to self-regulation, and manifesting good, positive outcomes. They begin with your knowledge and awareness of the pliability of thought, emotion, and energy. Most importantly, energy and your ability to govern it in accordance with your need and desired outcome.

Energy is the capability that sources the change. It's the catalyst for momentum. Thought and emotion are the relevant tools in the process, and matching the frequency of the desired outcome is the necessity.

Let's shed a little science on this thing to help bring it together a bit more intellectually but not too much. In the end, it's all about feeling, energy, and frequency.

Energy is defined as the capacity or power to perform an act. Essentially your emotional, feeling energy exerted through thought (mental energy) has the ability to produce a thing, a response, an action, or consequence.

The human brain is made up of three main parts: the cerebrum, cerebellum, and brain stem. The cerebrum is the biggest part and is responsible for interpreting touch, vision, sound, speech, reasoning, emotions, and movement control.

The brain is also made up of atoms formed of protons and neurons in a cell. The neurons hold billions of nerve fibers (axons and dendrites) that are basically energetic components used to send signals. They send electrical triggers to the nerves throughout our bodies. This is a natural process trigger that requires energetic influence to produce any desired function of or in the mind and body.

The heart is the largest energy producing organ in the body. Subsequent to the brain, it affects all other components. The brain, being the conduit, converts the emotional heart energy into thought.

When you feel something in a certain way, the brain translates that feeling, giving power to a process.

We are energy producing beings. In fact, our whole universe is made up of the same types of energy. Energy produces a thing, matter, form, or substance. Energy correlates with the object of its pull and produces an action, a function, an outcome, or some result; but energy is neither created nor destroyed. It just…is, waiting for stimulation or manipulation to advance its flow. Energy changes form all around us based on manipulation, but its existence is infinite. Energy is and has always been. Energy is everything, everywhere, and is one impetus in the scheme of specific, collaborative conduits, by which something materializes.

Emotions have energy that derive from the heart or a feeling of strong emotion. Even sound has energy. The energy that sound produces is vibration and is the premise for how our thought energies, converted to sound through spoken words, create a vibratory frequency that is powerful enough to affect our very atmosphere.

Everything that today is—which has become a manifested reality—started with the energy of emotion activating a thought process. Even when you go back to the beginning of our existence, our universe, our being. We began as a thought in the mind of our Creator, who then exercised that thought, converted it into energy, the energy of vibration, through the word that was spoken, bringing us and our universe into a realized, materialized existence.

Vibration, mixed with the power of intense emotional energy in thought and feeling, inspiring deliberate action in the form of spoken word, with the intensity of emotional energy, changes the external vibrational frequency of our very atmosphere. Even the molecules in the air we breathe are energy.

Again, everything is energy, and we are powerful creators, given the responsibility to do something here. To be accountable to and for this earthly dominion we have been given.

We, who are made in the image and likeness of God, Source, Creator, Infinite Intelligence—we have been endowed innately with the same power to create on this playground called earth.

Can you believe this, or are you still thinking inside the box you've been in your whole life? Before moving on, please pause and consider how that "box" thinking has been working for you.

Would you like to step out?

Let's talk about matter a bit. Matter is defined as that which materializes. It is the result of, or what, is produced after focused momentum and vibration align in frequency. Matter is the "stuff" of the universe and everything in it that makes up a physical thing. Whatever is real, tangible, has mass, and takes up space.

Focused energy has the potential to produce that which we have focused on. With a mixture of momentum, belief, faith in our belief, and strong emotion or feeling which drives the frequency of our vibration, powerful energy is produced, affecting the atmosphere.

Our work is to align with the frequency of that which we desire. The mode or method of the creation is not our concern, nor should it be a source of anxiety. We just need to be aligned with the frequency of the vibration, the energy in the belief of our desired outcome. See it, believe it, feel it, declare it, and expect it.

The potency of our energetic vibration and frequency affects our conscious awareness, reprogramming our subconscious mind to begin to create a complete change not only for the *course* of our lives, but for what our lives begin to produce. It's all so extremely exciting, and it's the substance of deliberate creating.

There is so much about our minds, our bodies, our human make up that is still undiscovered and untapped. We are now just beginning to awaken. Barely touching the surface of who we are and our innate capabilities. Evolving into the dynamic beings we were created to be because we dare to push past mediocre theories and sometimes contradictory theologies.

You've been asking for more knowledge, tried many formulas, methods, etc., not being satisfied or fulfilled.

Somehow stuck in or on what you were taught or conditioned to accept growing up.

Many of us are eager to experience new, pushing past the boundaries of the norm, daring to explore the intricacies that form our inner makeup. Eager to open up to all the universe has for us. Desirous of living our lives on the next level, without guilt, remorse, or feeling a sense of condemnation because we want to know more.

We are breaking free of rigid, regimented teaching meant to control and suppress. We realize and answer the call of that beckoning, the pull to Higher Conscious, and being made more fully aware of our intricate design as stated in the biblical reference found in the book of Psalms.

"I am fearfully and wonderfully made, and of this my soul is fully conscious."
(PSALMS 139:14, AMPLIFIED BIBLE)

In knowing this timeless truth, how could we not be compelled to ask the questions that begin to answer exactly *how* we are fearfully and wonderfully made? Or to wonder, based on that same premise of our wonderful beingness, *what* is our full potential and capability in the universe, in the world? It's what we are here for. To discover this life, who we are, what we are made of, and what we are here to create. An exciting adventure of discovery awaits. There are no limits except the ones that we place upon ourselves.

Therefore, it is vitally important that we check the vibrational output that we are emitting. This vibration can be either negative or positive; it depends on your thought vibration.

Stated earlier in this text, vibration was defined as energy that is converted to a vibration by sound. Vibration can also be created by the level or intensity of emotion put behind a thought. Vibration has a frequency, and that frequency's momentum is governed by the energy that it is given.

Newton's First Law of physics basically says that every object persists in its state of rest or uniform motion in a straight line, unless it is compelled to change that state by forces impressed upon it. This is momentum in physics.

Philosophically speaking, how much thought and emotion given to a thing can determine its momentum? Because energy is basically a force. It influences momentum and can be increased or decreased by the intensity of the energy exerted upon it.

For instance, consider a thought about a negative situation that you experienced. You produce a thought in your mind about it, and perhaps it causes some offense, so you have an emotional response. That thought about the situation, perceived as negative or offensive, begat a strong emotion which then resulted in negative, momentous energy.

Most of us would continue to replay the incident in our head, replaying how we felt, what we could have said, should have said, or done in our defense. All the while becoming more and more emotionally agitated (negative momentum) about the situation as we focused thought on it. Energy from that thought and the buildup of emotion behind it is the momentum. Negative, momentous energy is fueled, and now you are on that frequency. What your focused thought and emotions are on will manifest in your reality, affecting everything else going on in the day because of negative, vibratory energy being emitted.

When you think a thought with strong negative emotion, most often it will result in a reactionary response or action. Either you're pissed off at the world and show it, react with a stank attitude affecting your relationships, binge eat, get drunk, self-medicate, or you do something even worse to try and relieve this contrary momentum. This action leads to another then another, into a downward spiral that affects everything around you. This is the created reality you manifested.

"For every action there is an equal and opposite reaction"

– NEWTON'S THIRD LAW

Get off the frequency of negative vibration.

Since every action produces an equal and opposite reaction, why not deliberately change that energy? Choose a different emotion, deliberately. Choose not to react to a situation by default and learned behavior. Shift your energy by changing your emotional perspective and not forming an immediate, negative, emotionally driven opinion or response about the circumstance or situation but staying neutral. Controlling your thought energy by choosing to respond differently. Focusing emotional energy to see the experience as just that—an experience that you have the power to make negative, positive, neutral, or nothing. How much energy do you want to give it, and in what direction do you want that energy to unfold? Immediately begin to feel and think of how you want the experience to play out. Manipulate the energy into a deliberate, intentional, focused outcome that derives a benefit *For*, not against, the overall good.

IV

Be the Change You Want to See

"When you want something, all the universe conspires in helping you to achieve it"

–Paul Coelho

———ഝഝ———

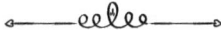

What an exciting revelation obtaining clarity out of obscurity can be if our perspective will allow it. Considerations of things outside of our daily resolve open a doorway to expansion. Expansion outside of the box. Powerful awakenings of the mind emerge when we consider a broader spectrum of the endless possibilities that lie before us. We are powerful creators. I cannot say this enough.

We have to say it until we believe it.

There is evidence all around you of this ability. Just look at your very own life and consider all that you have created. Really look, be still in this moment, and consider *your created life*.

How does it look to you, beloved? Are you happy with the outcome thus far? Anything you want to change or affect going forward? Or maybe you would like to enhance or tweak what is currently manifesting.

You can.

Change, adjust, upgrade, whatever. It starts with you.

We have been given so much freedom, autonomy, and creative genius, we can affect our lives in any way we choose.

Remember that thought processes, vibration, and thought energy also aid in our ability to create change. These are all tools in beginning that process and helping change come to fruition, giving us the results we want in our lives. It's all so extremely exciting when you really begin to grasp the concept of your being able to create the life you want. You are meant to take this life that you have been given and live it to the fullest. Whatever that looks like for you.

The Creator, God, Yahweh, Source, Infinite Intelligence, Allah (only One Creator, many names) provided a level playing field abundant with every resource imaginable. This includes you, appointed as co-creator, being planted on this earth, existing during these times, with daily opportunity to observe and consider whether or not you will capitalize on faith, conscious awareness, inspired action and make manifest the desires of your heart. Or are you good letting circumstances kick your ass by your lack of courage in asserting who you are as a *DIVINELY sourced* human?

...*What Do You Want?*

Be the change you want to see. Be it. Right now.

What do you see when you close your eyes? Think about it, feel the intense desire with your innermost heart and soul. What do you see? How do you see and feel yourself Being, Living, Loving, Thriving?

Be aware of your desire. Be grounded in knowing there are no limits or boundaries to what you can create besides the boundaries and limits you place in your own mind.

For us to be the change we want to see we must:

>> Acknowledge where we are.

>> Be surrounded with the thought and feeling of our desired change.

>> Practice being surrounded in that change as if it were already done. Walk in our desired temperament, conscious awareness, and energy, relative to who and how we want things to be.

>> Write our vision.

Acknowledging where you are needs to be priority. Present reality, where we are in the *NOW*, commands its consideration and respect. The present moment is fleeting, yes, but it gives us the premise on which to build our blueprint for forward movement and cultivation of the change. All of our past experiences, interactions, relationships, and decisions were based on some sort of belief about the situation. The energy and emotion behind that belief then formulated an idea that was brought to life, effected by an energetic process (*your powerful thoughts and responses in the form of energy*), driven by momentum, ultimately producing a living derivation of your current existence. That current existence being realized in the circumstances and situations we find ourselves dealing with today, and every day.

We may be seeing this place, this situation, this current reality and scratching our heads, wondering how we got here. But in essence the truth is, we arrived here by default instead of with Deliberate intent. Reactively responding and unconsciously effort-*ing* against the flow instead of proactively, consciously, with controlled awareness, recognizing and understanding the contrast and its actual role in aiding with and for our good.

Look at where you are and see it as an example of what default creating looks like. The Universe, in this context, is providing an opportunity for you to learn from and understand the difference between default and deliberate creating. An opportunity, to harness the art and power of deliberate thought and focused energy intentionally tailored to your desired change.

You are blessed with the power to effect a different outcome. It's what you are here for. On purpose. For purpose.

Be intentional.

The Creator has placed us here with free will and decision-making power. You are Not a damn puppet. There are no strings attached (literally and metaphorically). Do, Be the change you want to see.

Practice being surrounded by the desired change as if it were already done. Do not be conformed to this world and what it may look like in this moment. This moment is fleeting and will not last. Just as the world in its orbit is continually rotating and, in this rotation, the sun sets and rises, climates change, we experience night and day; so it is with the thing you see right now. It is not eternal but temporal.

Be transformed by the knowledge of your renewed thinking and smile because this condition you are seeing now is solely for your consideration. It is an opportunity to make a determination, to decide whether or not you are going to let it destroy you, kill your dream, your goals, your love. Or will you roll with it, allow it to pass, provide clarity, growth, and, most importantly, a life lesson that will be molded *into* use *for* your ultimate good.

Everything is working for your good. But now, with conscious awareness of this, you should feel moved with excitement and enthusiasm. Inspired. Knowing that through your integral participation, with deliberate focus, realizing and believing in your innate power, and commandment of the energy around you…not only is change inevitable, but positive change is possible.

So how do you want it to go?

You may be thinking to yourself, what does it mean to "practice being surrounded in the desired change"? Practicality is necessary here, but so is imagination because being surrounded in the desired change requires both thought processes.

For instance, in your now, in your current reality, you see, you observe what is. In your imagination, you see, think, feel what can be. What you desire.

We have already addressed how powerful thought is and how the energy of thought and emotions creates a momentum. If you can begin to practice, even in your now situation, visualizing your life, your attitude, your circumstances, as *you want them to be*, this begins to stir up that momentum of creative, deliberate intent.

One cannot help but smile or start to feel good when you begin imagining things as you want them to be.

Ok, I hear the naysayers now: "Sounds like a bunch

of malarkey," or "That's unrealistic and you are trying to escape what is real and live in an imaginary existence that will result in nothing."

Lies.

Faith or belief in a thing starts the manifestation. All things that were ever created started with imagining that thing coming to fruition. Without thought, without a little dreaming, without taking time to envision what you want or see yourself having, how can you ever even begin to bring it to pass? There's no premise.

When you begin to take time each day to invest in your thoughts, specifically and on purpose. Then feeling good about what you are thinking on, giving that thought emotion as it develops momentous energy. Don't you think that what you dwell on intently will eventually gain life and manifest?

Oh my goodness, it's a powerful thing. Your positive energy on thoughts of your desired change Will create momentum; momentum will promote a desire to create, and that desire will become inspired action. You just move on the inspiration as it is given in confirmation of your thought. You will begin to ask the Universe for the plan to unfold. As you are given the layout, your actions will confirm the vision, and you will see that shit happen in your life and be fucking amazed.

Your imagination outlines the blueprint. Literally Ask for the plan, the course of action, and think on it every day. Feel yourself in it, practice and repeat the feeling of it until it consumes you to the point that You know in your deepest knowing that what you have asked, imagined, visualized *is* Done and you are just in a place of waiting-allowing the tangible evidence of its existence.

I want you to practice thinking from the perspective of already having obtained. Think it, feel it, know it. Be it. Whatever your it is.

With all these fine words and spirited motivations, you should be pumped, and the wheels of imagination should be turning. Glimpses and mental imageries of your most delicious desires should be flashing through your mind, waiting for your yes and permission to be fueled with your practiced, deliberate considerations.

Mm mmm, that's good, baby.

So, with that said, let's start giving these thoughts life. How about we "write the vision and make it plain." Now don't flake out on me; it's not like I said,

"Lets write our goals." *Ewww*. Something about the word goals has always made me uncomfortable. Icky even, like undertaking a burdensome task that makes my chest hurt and heart palpitate incessantly. But no, this is not a goal-setting task. Unless, of course, you prefer the more technical term, then think of it as such.

However, writing a vision entails something passionate. It's more...personal. You are not tasking or efforting. You are creating your story as you see it. Drawing the blueprint to savor, be mindful of, refer to as needed, and build upon. Vision *is your realized plan of creation* in written form.

Writing your vision is a sort of faith exercise. It's what your faith will be exercised from and; by virtue of, strengthened to attract the very thing its purposed intent is focused towards.

> *"Now faith is the assurance [title deed, confirmation] of things hoped for [divinely guaranteed], and the evidence of things not seen [the conviction of their reality—faith comprehends as fact what cannot be experienced by the physical senses]."*
> (HEBREWS 11:1, AMPLIFIED BIBLE)

If you don't have the faith to believe in the possibilities of change or that you possess the power to create and live your best life, how can you have vision? There is nothing to support it. Get some faith to fuel your dreams, awaken your creative intelligence, and be conscious of and prepared for inspired action.

When you're ready......

Write your vision:

1. Grab your journal (you know—the one you used with Chapter II) and your favorite pen.

2. Find a quiet place. Uncluttered, if possible. Your favorite creative space. Outside, inside, wherever you feel free, relaxed.

   Sit quietly in this place for a moment; you can actually refer back to the meditation exercise in Chapter I and take ten-to-fifteen minutes to quiet your mind and get centered before you begin your vision writing. Or do the meditation immediately after you complete the vision exercise to connect your concepts to the subconscious.

3. If you choose to begin without meditation, just sit quietly, being still and coming to a state of calm attentiveness. Begin to think about all the things you want to do, be, experience, and accomplish. Just let your mind go. Dream big. Imagine and see yourself

being, doing, having these things. Picture yourself as the actor, producer, and videographer on the opposite side of a video camera filming your life. What do you see? What does your life look like? What are the feelings and emotions you experience as these visions are taking place on the projection screen of your life? From the most minute thing to the most decadent extravagance. Have fun with this. Just let your mind indulge itself in these deliberate thoughts until you are filled with the confirmation of "I can have all of this."

4. Open your journal and reflect upon the things you just visualized. What stands out to you?

    Write it down.

    You might begin just intuitively writing down lists of words or phrases that stand out to you: more money, wealth, community, charity, strong relationships, stability. Any words or phrases that resonate with your subconscious, evoking an intense feeling or emotion.

Or you might just start writing your vision as a story of your life. For example, "I see myself running a nonprofit organization. I am helping so many people. I feel happy and accomplished. I am receiving so much support both financially and professionally." Or "I am making an extra $10,000 a month. I am traveling around the world. I see myself walking along the shore of a beautiful beach in Santorini. I am purchasing my first home; it's located in…" Just draft your story as you see it. Again, don't be concerned about the format.

5. If you'd like to set a timer for fifteen, twenty, or thirty minutes, you can do that. This exercise is something you want to set aside time to do regularly. Make time for it. Don't get tangled up in the intricacies or formatting of this exercise. As you practice taking time to write and review your vision, it will develop into an arrangement that is clarified to your standard. Being the change that you want to see requires process, practice, and commitment. Begin today.

"Success is the sum of small efforts repeated day in and day out."

–R. COLLIER

V

Discipline and Time Management

"Lack of direction, not lack of time, is the problem. We all have twenty-four-hour days."

–Zig Ziglar

———— ꞏꞏꞏ ————

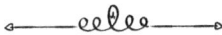

To support balance in our lives, we must first be aware of now—time and space; our ability to govern them with respect to our needs and our vision. Everything is pliable. Getting order in our day to day is as easy as setting boundaries in and to what we allow. What you allow access into your life tends to pervade it incessantly.

Therefore, it is especially important to protect this space, to protect your time so that order can be maintained. Without order you are relegated to chaos, and through chaos, you open yourself up to discord and stress.

With all that we are faced with in our daily activities, why on earth would we want to deliberately subject ourselves to any thing, person, substance or situation that would further deplete us? We can set boundaries by limiting what we allow to filter through our personal lives so that we are grounded enough to manage our external day-to-day. Balance begins internally. Whatever is going on on the inside eventually bleeds out into our external lives.

If there are never any boundaries set, then our peace of mind, direction, and purpose could be resigned to impassiveness. Causing dreams or goals to fade to nothing.

There needs to be clear boundaries set up that check and regulate the flow of things coming in and out of your life. You have choices; you have the power to make decisions and order or construct the life you want.

There are those that thrive on chaos because there may be some level of functionality in it for them, especially if it provides a challenge to overcome. Finding solutions can be like an adrenaline rush as you take action to solve issues or make conditions right. Even a little chaos is apt to produce elevated levels of motivation to action, by reaction to the prodding stimuli. However, for others it is a peace stealer, a prescription for stagnation and anxiety leading to a feeling of lost control.

Many people constantly speak of the need for time management. For many the remedy is writing lists of things to do or calendaring their entire life's agenda by day, minute, or hour, all to secure some semblance of order in the daily grind. These actions are not at all uncommendable, but what is your purpose behind them? What is your motive in creating the agenda? Are you compelled to write a list of things that need to get done because you can't remember to do them? Are you calendaring and creating an agenda of things that need to be done based on an unfavorable condition in your life that you feel is out of control? How has it helped you when creating them with that perspective? Have you noticed any changes as a result of those efforts, or are you still experiencing complete inefficiency of your household, finances, personal or professional life?

Instead of making tasks easier, as the intent of the calendaring was meant to capture, have we not simply just created a neat little numbered, timed, dated, categorized list of sporadic confusion in a more concise and categorized manner? Looking good on the outside and on paper, giving the appearance of a life well maintained, organized and scheduled to the hour, on the hour. The only problem is that, every time we look at it, a feeling of overwhelming anxiety ensues at the daunting tasks written out before us.

It's not the list of busy things that is the issue. It's the mindset and emotional compartmentalization we feel when considering the mode of execution. How are you looking at your list of busy things? What is your emotion?

Name it. Is it anxiety? Is it a feeling of "Oh my goodness," or "WTF? How am I going to get all this done?"

Can you even for a moment consider releasing some of your control so rigidly drawn out in your to do lists? Can you Stop? Breathe. Consider that you are Not out of control; it's just that sometimes all of our *doing* causes us to fight against the natural flow of circumstances, situations, or seasons of our lives.

Our tendency is to take some immediate actions to remedy or try and control the situation, which can result in our being inundated and drowning as we grab hold of shallow tasks, agendas, and things to Do, in an attempt to find an anchor. Yet we have not First taken time to consider Higher Conscious directive that will be imparted to us when we take time to go within and practice mindful meditation. Then, tailored solutions and inspired directives are given to us based upon our unique individual qualities and strengths, exclusively known by Source, embedded in our psyche, awaiting download.

Our first action should be getting tuned in and tapping into our connection to Source, in an effort to receive divine guidance and ascertain the best approach of how to flow with this thing or *things to do,* in a manner that affords us the least resistance to our productivity. This should be our first item on the "to do list".

Instead, we often forego this due diligence, perpetuating a spinning of the wheels cycle of repetitive doing, expending *good energy* only to our disadvantage. Can you just simply tap into the congruency of alignment Universe is directing you in and allow things to unfold in a revelatory way that makes your doing purposeful?

Let me clarify here. I am not anti-agenda or anti-calendaring. Nor do I abhor the proactivity in doing. Personally I'm obsessed with doing; but just doing for the sake of doing can become robotic, leave us unfulfilled, mechanical, and may even exacerbate stress. Going through the motions, mindlessly checking off a list of things to do, without any connection to true purpose. Oftentimes this type of unconscious doing can be a scapegoat, avoidance from dealing with something else pervading your life that you don't want to or cannot deal with at the time. Being urged by the mind's incessant goading or suggestion that there is a dire need for fulfillment of tasks can become an added source of stress, i.e., "*Don't think, just doooo.*"

The solution is to find alignment by seeking guidance from Source so that direction is downloaded to our higher conscious. Going within and manifesting without. Not being ruled by the conscious mind's practiced reaction to what *IS*, attempting to affect control intellectually by randomly tasking and creating to do lists to get on top of the situation. But instead, being introspective, discovering a better understanding of your why and gaining clearer guidance to your solution with clarity. You want clarity in your agenda.

You are not your mind. You are soul and spirit having this life experience in a human body. The mind is a part of you, as well as your will, and your emotions. The setup of this threesome is constructed to be utilized with deliberate exercise of the attributes bestowed upon you by the Creator—with an expectation of specific, conscious, and purposed use. Do not be ruled by the mind, disconnected from higher consciousness. Train your mind to be still and connect to Source, to your soul self, your inner being.

As you begin to incorporate the exercises provided throughout this book, you will feel a sense or desire to act. I encourage you to act on the inspiration that is given. It is expected that, as you begin to awaken to higher conscious and to the guidance of Source you will become more aware of the power in your thoughts. Based on your newly expressed desires, natural inspiration, and clarity, your *purposed* agenda will become more prevalent. The key is to be aware of your ability to control this flow of inspiration. Do not become overwhelmed with the flood of ideas and the plans to perfect them as they start presenting themselves in your subconscious and seeping through to conscious reality.

Chaos does not have to ensue; anxiety does not have to preclude success and innovation. This flow of ideas and innovation is exactly what you want. Embrace it, have an awareness of it, and create your agenda by it.

Having a mindless list of items on a calendar or a to-do list is fruitless unless you want to use it as a reminder of sorts; but does true creation solely consist of a list of to-do items that can quickly become, rigid, robotic and extremely task oriented?

Our day-to-day activities already consist of a pretty regimented, sometimes over-scheduled, and very often-mundane routine. Inspiration allows us to escape the claustrophobic confines of that box and tap into what we truly aspire to create in our lives. Consciously, deliberately executing clear pathways for specific outcomes gained from taking the time to go within, instead of random intellect based on our mind's drive or the adoption of someone else's prescribed process of tasking in an effort to gain control of what we think is out of control.

Inspired thought process through introspection and connection to higher conscious helps us to develop understanding of our now and aids in the conceptual creativity of solution derived from the benefit of higher consciousness's connection to Source. That same Source who knows the ins, outs, and intricacies of any given situation and the method by which it can be resolved most effortlessly, with the least amount of resistance. Connecting to Infinite Intelligence through higher conscious makes our agendas purposeful, less stressful, clear, and concise. It's like we have tapped into the source of inside information and knowing, allowing our soul perspective and insight to properly direct our tool (the mind) to develop a plan that unfolds with clarity so we come to know exactly how to move, what to do, and how to create true agendas based on that understanding and connection.

When you consider the time that we are given on this earth, what a waste it is when you consider the routines we tend to construct on our little calendars, our phones, or refrigerator list of "things to do." Are these things really helping us live? Or are they simply a source or system used to help us feel normal, productive, like we are *doing something*, yet all the while only making us more robotic and desensitized to our inner selves?

What is the purpose behind our doings? Are these doings for purpose, on purpose, or just something to *doooooo*? Do we have balance?

We must become more aware and in tune with who we are and what we truly want to be happening in our lives so we can make our *do's* significant. I believe that with awareness and clarity being our endeavor, our "tasking" and to do lists will be more fulfilling. Do everything with purpose, not in the functionality of *just doing* as a crutch to make us feel productive. Seriously, let's Be productive inspirationally so that it means something.

This perspective is the other side of that anxiety or overwhelming feeling we get when looking at our great agendas, calendaring, and to-do lists. This is the opposite side of that coin from feeling a sense of stress at all that we have written out and scheduled in our lives. When our lists and agendas evolve into the stories we write for our lives or are transformed from mere agendas on a calendar into our visions and plans, there is a sense of connection. Actual purpose is developed in the effort. We are connected to and stirred by our creation. Thereby alleviating the stress resulting from overexerting ourselves in the doing of things for the sake of just doing, routinely or under compulsion.

Get order in your life but not order that is stifling. Get order that is balanced, aligned, and freeing. Order that comes with an awareness that we are not just our minds or the rampant thinking of our minds. Being aware that our mind is a collective tool in conjunction with our will, emotions, and in connection with higher conscious.

Drawing from Higher Conscious or heightened awareness provides direction through the path of least resistance, allowing us the ability to exercise and bring to fruition the purpose of our souls' deepest, innermost desires, to which we were created and put on this earth to carry out.

We are not robots living out a list of things to do to keep us functioning. We are here to live. Please understand and grasp this. Live, live on purpose not by default.

VI

Little Victories Lead to Great Success

> *"The man who moves a mountain begins by carrying away small stones."*
> –CONFUCIUS

> *"Building upon successes one victory at a time. No matter how small"*
> –APRYL K.

———— eeeee ————

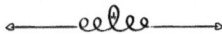

*D*o not ever discount the feats or accomplishments you have made that others may trivialize. Your life is big. Every victory, every obstacle that you have overcome, speaks volumes. It does not matter who may try to discount your victories; you know what you had to do to come through, to overcome every obstacle that you were faced with. What it took to keep your sanity, your livelihood, or even your will to live.

All those little victories were the precursor and preparation, a sort of boot camp course that, if you survived, would land you another opportunity to get it right. Today your lessons have prepared you for purpose.

Now is the time, the opportunity, to build upon those earlier victories and start focusing on your future success.

We must begin to consider those victories. The things that we have accomplished or survived truly are an attestation of our ability to overcome anything deemed an obstacle to our intended destination or accomplishment. These small victories are part of the contributory details that complement our future plans and give evidence that "Hey, if I came through that and still accomplished what

I intended, then I can successfully steer my way through this as well."

They serve as a guide, instructions, key points, and lessons for us to use going forward. Even our presumed failures serve a purpose in preparation for future successes. It all depends on how you look at them in retrospect.

Some people set out to accomplish something, end up failing at that goal, and simply throw in the towel at that point, presumably defeated, never looking back on the intended goal or endeavor, stuck in fear at the remembrance of past failure. That's when they let go of dreams that were very strongly desired. The problem with this is that failure should not have been the end of the pursuit. It may be that, even in your own experience with a seemingly failed or failing situation, you found yourself on the very edge of success but allowed the encroachment of trepidatious thoughts of past failures stop you in your tracks. Had you just gotten right back up and tried again or pushed yourself a little bit further, you might have discovered that your victory was right on the other side.

Maybe even if you had gone back to the drawing board and revisited the plans or reached out to that friend, family member, or lover, reconciliation, accomplishment, and/or your desired outcome might have been realized.

There are so many stories of famous people who were rejected, denied, or repeatedly failed at their efforts. The only difference between them is that they decided they would not give up. Their dream or desire was just too much to let go. Sometimes you must want it so bad that it becomes your obsession and you do not let anything throw you off the course of its obtainment.

For example, Thomas Edison. Everyone knows he invented the light bulb. But did you know that he failed over 1000 times at perfecting his invention before it actually worked? Just imagine. Had he not pushed himself one more time or tweaked his data or calculations and tried one more time, we would be deprived of electricity and still be living in the gotdamn dark ages, lighting fires and lanterns and shit. Barred from the blessing of technological advances that electricity affords us today.

I should not have to go into detail about all of the other great people that, in spite of obstacles, continued to move forward with their dreams and ideals, only to meet success by the diligence of their endeavors. Abraham Lincoln, Mahatma Gandhi, Martin Luther King, and so many others. I am sure their failures seemed huge and, at times, insurmountable. The remarkable thing is that, amid their failures, there were also small victories along the way that encouraged more steps toward their vision and purpose. Every small step that resulted in a victory was their catalyst to continue and eventually gain huge victories that affected a multitude of others.

Perhaps your vision is not as grandiose or your reach not as broad, but you are here for purpose. Every small victory, every dusting off of yourself—getting back up and trying again is so powerful. You have no idea what effect your tenacity and follow-through is having on the world. We are all co-contributors to this universe, no matter how small or large our sphere of influence. Your success is important; that is why you have been able to come through the things you have come through. To prove that you *Can* and to also prove to someone else that *they Can*.

Our small victories lead to greater success than we even realize; they are the steppingstones to our next levels. They are proof that anything is possible, a call to challenge ourselves, dream bigger dreams, and get after it.

So what does that mean? I mean get after it and live on purpose. Be about your business. Stop adjusting yourself to tempestuous conditions. Swaying back and forth with every wave of adversity or contrast. Scared to move forward and push against it a little for the sake of your vision. Acting in trepidation, desperately adjusting your sails to accommodate adversity's demand, or simply conceding defeat at its surge, only rebounding slightly, enough to gather energetic resources to simply survive the next round—not on purpose, but by default, giving away your goal.

Living on purpose is the opposite of default living.

Do not be naïve or ignorant in thinking that there is no contrast or that somehow every obstacle becomes obsolete because you have decided to purposefully focus and pursue your endeavors at all costs.

Hellll no.

In fact, as a test of your true sentiment, you may find that life may allow you to encounter even more contrasting situations—or, as I like to refer to them, opportunities.

However, the intent, knowing, and power of purpose affords a solidarity of mind in holding steadfastly to our belief in the thing that we endeavor to accomplish. We cultivate a healthy abhorrence to anything that resembles a concession to our efforts because we begin to realize and accept that we are more than conquerors.

Living on purpose involves deliberate thought and a deliberate, conscious, decision-making process. It involves conscious thought, invested time, and some energy. Notice, I said energy and not effort-*ing*. Yes, there is a difference.

Because we can shape our outcomes and there is so much that is available to us, why not live on purpose? Of course, discovering our purpose is key, and that also comes with some deliberate action.

You probably have already begun this process, although your intention may not have been deliberate. Life has a way of steering us into the direction of destiny, without any propelling actions on our part. In fact, sometimes in that steering, we find ourselves escaping unscathed, barely by the skin of our teeth. I call this living by default, a word that I'm sure you may be tired of hearing, as it has been repeatedly referenced throughout this entire book. Its emphasis or repetitive presence is because we need to understand that we do not have to live a life by default. Every small victory or step in the direction of your goals is walking out intended purpose in your life.

Up till now, yes, you may have been practicing default living, but you are now being made aware of your prowess in deliberately creating a life that you love. This whole time, even by default, you were in training mode as the Universe found ways to rock your path here and there, challenge you in some aspect or area of your life that forced a reaction, a move, or other action. Again, by default. Nonetheless, habitually, you rose to the occasion and met the challenge, whether by being dragged into it responding by fight or flight response trying to escape it or find a solution or way out, and that thing passed over. You survived. Small victory, but you realized you could get through it, even if only by the skin of your teeth. .

Now how about taking this realization and kicking it up a notch by being more deliberate in the planning of the direction that you want things to go by making clear conscious decisions toward where you see yourself. What you see yourself doing. Visualizing the outcome of every circumstance in the manner toward which you see it unfolding for you. Finding your purpose. Deliberately practicing, manifesting your desired outcome in any situation, as opposed to just letting things happen and accepting them no matter what it looks like.

I honestly believe there is more to it than that, and my intention is to broaden your thinking so that you begin to grasp the infallible truth that you are a powerful creator. If you want a specific type of life, you want to accomplish your dreams, your goals, and the things you have only dreamed about but never dared to share with anyone, then do that. I dare you. That's your purpose. That is the thing you are meant to do. Yes...That—the biggest dream, the biggest goal, the thing that, when you think about it, you get full of tingles and teary eyes Just because you want it so badly but think it's silly, out of your reach, or not practical and seems like an impossibility. Noooo, that is your passion coming through on that thing, your soul indicator on purpose. You can do just that. I need you to believe that it is possible for you and that there are no limitations besides the ones you place in your own way.

How badly do you want it? Beginning this journey to purpose is not for the faint of heart or mind. It will require decisive tenacity on your part and an almost obsessive desire for that thing you want to achieve.

Those small victories on your way to your Now have more than prepared you for this place. Even if you start taking baby steps toward this vision. Even something as small as research, an inquiry, a class, a book on the topic. Take those steps because every small step you take toward purpose becomes bigger, bolder, and allows the Universe to clear the path for your next visualized step. The seed has been planted, and that thing will grow as long as you continue to feed it with faith and deliberate intent. Only this time around you have awareness of your capacity as co-creator; staying connected to higher conscious through mindfulness, prayer, or meditation with God, Source, Infinite Intelligence (one Creator, many names). When you step into your deliberate planning, the universe works with you and begins to reveal the specific path that you need to take to allow for those deliberate opportunities, setups, right-place-right-time experiences, and delightful surprises that align with your purpose.

You must block out the naysayers, the doubters, and those who only know you by what you have done or experienced in the past. In fact, protect your vision and your purpose and be careful revealing all your plans and details with everyone; not everyone is on the same path, and not everyone is ready to support you in this pursuit. Use wisdom when discussing your endeavors. You will know who to share with and who not to until the timing is appropriate. Treasure your dream and allow it to develop.

If you ever get stuck or start to feel overwhelmed, remember to reflect back on the small victories you've come through, knowing that they were, in essence, the training grounds necessary for teaching you how to overcome obstacles. Valuable outcomes and necessary lessons that if looked at with the right perspective, confirm the Universe is not against you but is helping you grow up to this point, and is desirous of your success. You have enough experience with default living conditions and outcomes to now be more deliberate in your future intentions. Appreciate your small victories, for they are the stones that build the bridges for greater pathways. Your future is bright, and you are so ready.

VII

Gratitude

"Gratitude is the healthiest of all human emotions. The more you express gratitude for what you have, the more likely you will have even more to express gratitude for."

–ZIG ZIGLAR

————꧁꧂————

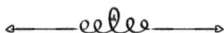

When all else fails, be grateful. Gratitude is the catalyst that opens the door for more, propels you to higher heights. You may not realize it, but the moment you turn to gratefulness in response to a negative situation, you are affecting the atmosphere. Changing the momentum. Showing, feeling, expressing gratitude is powerful; it causes a shift and speaks directly to negativity and stops its deceptive antics dead in their tracks. Gratitude is like a weapon you employ in the travail of contrasting life battles. It is a deliberate change in perspective. It's like saying:

"No. I refuse to succumb to that which appears in my Now as unfavorable to my goals or what I think I should have or be experiencing in this moment. Passionately believing that Everything is working out for my good, I am choosing to shift and direct focus on all the good that is around me. Everything in my present circumstance that Is good, that Is a blessing, that I Can be thankful for. I Will focus on that, while everything else serves its purpose, yields to my sword of gratitude, and conforms to serve my intended good."

Being thankful is powerful. For one, you are acknowledging the wonderful aspects of your life that afford you opportunity, life, living, substance.

If you are not able to look around you, observe, think of, or feel anything that is good, then I'm sorry, but I don't know if simply reading this book and applying its principles will be of any benefit. An inability to find even one tiny semblance of something to be grateful for, even if it is just the obvious fact you are alive right now, implies a complete dissatisfaction with life. Most assuredly diminishing your vitality.

There is so much to be grateful for; I am talking even the smallest thing. The most miniscule, little thing to one person is so big to another. You are not comparing your level of gratitude with another though; I just want you to consider gratefulness in its simplest, most tangible form.

Do you think about your life? Do you consider that today you woke up in your bed, alive and well, limbs intact, vision intact, healthy, on your way to wholeness?

Did you ever stop to consider that someone did not, is not, or cannot?

Did you ever stop to consider the intricate design of your human body and how it runs every day…on…what? Grace maybe? Nonetheless you are alive today, reading this book; even that is enough to be grateful for. If you cannot think of anything else to be grateful for, say thanks for that.

I assume all this gratefulness talk may seem frivolous to some. We want the crux of this process, the goal that will afford us an advantage, a strategy to get to where we are going. Well the greatest of these processes is gratefulness, being mindful and aware of all that we have been provided. Do you recognize the beauty and graciousness in the many life-sustaining, life-giving, freebies in our world today? Or might I also draw attention to those aesthetically pleasing natural wonders created for our pleasure and enjoyment. The fact that we didn't even have to work for most of it—should amplify the message that the Creator desires to freely give us *all* things. More tangible evidence of this fact is supported by the breath of life we breathed throughout the night, which was sustained and continued into morning, allowing us to wake up and experience the gift of yet one more day.

If you cannot take time to appreciate even this and to be grateful for where you have come from, what you have come through, or even where you are now, how can or will the Universe be assured that you will be grateful for any future success or opportunity? Will you even appreciate it? Or is your capacity for more stifled and impossible to be realized exponentially because you lack the ability to grasp the importance of gratitude for what has already been given and realized in your here and now?

When you take time to recognize and be grateful for what is here and now, this consideration allows for the opportunity and expansion of more. This is what we want. We want our lives filled to the brim with abundance. Thinking of abundance in terms of material substance is only one representation of the multiplicity in this word. Abundance does not always connote acquisitiveness.

Broaden your imagination and consciousness so your vision encompasses all that abundance means for you. That includes the abundance of life. All areas of our lives. Our money, love, relationships, peace of mind, lifestyle, way of life, and living. We can have abundance in all those areas. This broader concept of abundance always equates to the true meaning of wealth in my humble opinion. What greater way to live a sustainable, healthy, happy life than in a life of abundance in all things? This is a well- rounded life full of wealth and all things that are good.

As you deeply consider having gratitude for all things—even the things we look at and think of as the most devastating and stifling, can you look back and see how those circumstances—depending on or irrespective of your perspective and response—actually contributed to your greater good in the end? Even if the only good that came out of it was the great lesson you learned that caused a shift in your way of thinking, doing, or being, it made you ask for change and set you on that path.

This is what I mean. This is the premise for gratefulness. Being able to look back on all the negative and finding some semblance of good in it. Finding the good, finding the lesson in obscurity, creates expansion, if we allow it. A wealthy, grateful life worth living abundantly.

So take time to enjoy your life and consider the things that truly make you happy. Do not allow your life to be stifled by any obstacles or the lack of gratitude. Your life is truly what you make it, and, again, there is so much to be grateful for, if you just take the time each day to be still and consider them.

You'll find, any negativity that might have put you in a different mindset will gradually dissipate, once you shift your focus to the many blessings in your life that you may have, in the past, taken for granted or just neglected to reflect upon. You will find that all the good that is showing up in your life now far outweighs the negative. Your change in perspective, which allows you to focus on all that good, will quickly change the trajectory of the current momentum.

Remember, "It's all energy and vibrational frequency."

Change the frequency, and you will change the direction of your emotions, thereby initiating an effect that will act as a catalyst in changing the dynamic of the energy around you. Nothing stays the same, and this too shall pass because change is constant.

You never have to stay in a feeling or emotion that is contrary to how you want to feel just because the current situation or circumstance, in its appearance, dictates that you should. You are not your circumstance or situation; it is just momentary contrast. You do not give it your good energy by becoming fearful and stressed about it; that's resistance. Observe it, be consciously aware of it, and recognize that it is passing through and will give way to balance if you can allow it. Allow the contrast to pass without resistance but don't accept or be intimidated by its presence.

Find and shift to an emotion of gratitude in believing that, even in this thing…all is working for your good. This will take intentional practice and repetition to stick, but eventually it will become set in your subconscious as the most immediate and proper way to respond to contrasting situations in your life that tend to drain you. On the other side of it all, you will see that contrast does not in any way minimize or diminish Divine purpose; it strengthens it along with your resolve to keep moving forward.

Be grateful.

VIII

The Best Part

"Decide what you want. Believe you can have it. Believe that you deserve it, and believe it is possible for you."
–Jack Canfield

"Be You. Do You. For You. First."
–Unknown

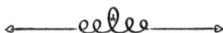

Love yourself. Love who you are. All of you. Even if you start out in a shitty mess full of stupid mistakes, bad choices, broken places, there is still good in you. You are Not a mistake. There is purpose in you. That is why you are still here. *You* must look at *you* and embrace everything that has shaped who you are today because that is where you are starting from, and this is okay. You have the tools you need to write a new story and let it be built upon where you have come from. You are a beautiful human even in your imperfections. It is possible that some of those attributes you consider negative are things that make up some of the greatness in you. You just need to take time and figure out what that was or is.

For instance, I have always been told that I am stubborn, hardheaded, and that I do not listen. I chose to recognize that this equates to "I Am tenacious, driven, strong, and not easily swayed by the opinion of others." Flip that old script and find how your negatives translate to the badass you really are. Use it to your advantage, Not your demise or the diminution of your self-esteem. The best part of any life is the culmination of events, circumstances, and situations that allow you to shape your best life. We all want to live, love, be loved, celebrated and prosperous. The trick is finding our flow and alignment with the universe and elevating our mind to meet the Creators expectations. Life consists of so many intricate details, and we—as very unique, individual beings—have the broad tapestry of a designed life story to share and tell, a tapestry that is intertwined with ups, downs, and sideways situations we have overcome.

There is nothing that can stop you from living your best life and being your absolute *best* you except You. There are absolutely no excuses that can justify why you cannot, so stop making them up and bringing them into your reality. We do not gauge *OUR* personal best by the standards a limited thinking society imposes by their lack of vision. There are some of *those* types, but few. I genuinely believe that the majority's desire for greater is predominant. It is just those slackers with limited ability to see past the bullshit who are still stuck and pushing an antiquated mentality.

Nonetheless, this is about you and where you want to take this story of your life. How do you want to build upon the principles, experiences, and revelations that have come into your awareness? How do you want to grow? What is your vision or idea of success? That is what matters. The tapestry of your life inadvertently weaves its way into and collides with others in a shared experience leading to wholeness and fulfillment—just a different path perhaps. In the end, we all come together and are able to realize that each of our experiences have meaning and are relatable.

Additionally, — maybe our newfound wisdom and awareness will motivate us to share our journey and encourage someone to start their own. Especially for those who have not yet awakened to the concept of living life on purpose, living a life above circumstance.

Not all of us are going to write books or become celebrities, movie stars, rock stars, or political figures, but setting examples and living out our elevation in any context in front of others, conservatively or quietly, is testimony enough. There are probably those in your circle or sphere of influence that draw their eyes to you as you begin to implement changes and endeavor to stop living by default. Some may notice the difference and want to know what it is about you that is bringing on all this good. You may not even be consciously aware that this is the case. Then there are those who you are aware of, those in your direct line of contact or sixth degree of separation. Perhaps you have seen or heard about someone in that group who may be struggling day-to-day, year-after-year, losing hope, giving up, sinking. Regarding the latter and considering our new found mindset, elevated thinking, successful application and results; it seems appropriate to be empathetic and inclined to share that knowledge, solely for the purpose of seeing someone achieve the same or even better.

The best part of an elevated life is that the enlightened awareness fills you up to overflowing so much, that the invisible energy in your *knowing* brims over, flows out and into the life of another. Our positive vibration becomes magnetic because we have a connection to one another that draws us to good energy, when we recognize it and can appreciate it without jealousy or envy.

When we feel so good about our lives and our shift in the direction and realization of our purpose, we inevitably become shining magnets on this earth, bright lights of enthusiasm that cannot be hidden; and when we love ourselves, we have an even bigger capacity to love others and express it in many different forms. Think creatively in this, outside the box. Try to be open to the right timing and opportunity. Everyone has their respective journey to awareness, and your chance encounter or interaction may be their start...

When you find your balance, it is okay if you feel moved or inspired to give a little. Somehow, somewhere; to pay it forward, so to speak. Giving back not only feels good but also perpetuates a good karmic cycle. What you give out or make happen for others comes right back to you in the same manner it was given or in the manner considered most appropriate by Source.

Oftentimes, when we are seeking the elevated life and on our journey to balance, wholeness, and living our best lives, we do not readily have the ability to give to anyone, and that's okay. Never feel incomplete or not enough, if your well is dry. There are times to be selfish. There are times to preserve energy because, if you don't, you're basically giving yourself out from an empty source, which further depletes you and helps no one.

Staying connected to the Source is the vitalization that replenishes. Daily mindfulness has the capacity to keep you full. Getting quiet, being still, and tapping into higher conscious at the start of your day. Taking care of *you* first and foremost helps to maintain your positivity and good energy as you move through your day. This also helps you to consider the course of action you want to take and allows you to set the tone of it.

Being deliberate in your initial thought process, considering all aspects of your life in your journaling and vision writing, also puts any unexpected contrast in perspective. Practicing mindfulness will make you more aware, more grounded, more prepared for all possibilities, and exactly how you will address any contrasting situations that may arise. Do not be resistant to the contrast but allow it as a passing concept, only to be observed and considered, knowing that with its presence there is opportunity for consideration that leads to the balancing out of your overall objective, because "*everything is always working out for you.*"

What you have, who you are, the strength and wisdom you have garnered along the way are a big deal; your life is big. The small victories of your life have brought you to this very place in time. No matter what it looks like in your now, that situation is not a contingent factor to where you are going; it is just the current sentiment, and it does not mean you have to accept it as a stumbling block that impedes your intended progress. Change your perspective. Use any weakness as an opportunity to learn where your strength lies. There is no failure; there is no defeat. It is only your mindset. That is your most formidable competitor. Change your thoughts; change your life.

My hope is that you are inspired to go forward and conquer not just the day, but your life. Knowing that you have everything to make what you deem good enough for you—a reality.

Dig deep and pull out that which drives and motivates you. Find your passion and let your soul speak. Get deliberate, write your vision; and the Universe will enlighten the path and show you the way. It will be in alignment with where you want and need to go. Trust your intuition, confident in the time you have spent quieting your mind and listening to the deepest part of you—as well as impartation from the Creator that you've got this—and all that you have faith to dream is possible. You have everything innately provided for you to thrive. It is in you.

So, get after it.

www.ingramcontent.com/pod-product-compliance
Lightning Source LLC
Chambersburg PA
CBHW052209270326
41931CB00011B/2281